DIETER'S LITTLE BOOK
OF WISDOM

By William W. Forgey, M.D.

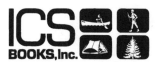

ICS BOOKS, Inc.
Merrillville, IN

Dieter's Little Book of Wisdom
Copyright © 1996 by William W. Forgey, M.D.
10 9 8 7 6 5 4 3 2 1

All rights reserved, including the right to reproduce this book or portions thereof in any form or by any means, electronic or mechanical, including photocopying, recording, unless authorization is obtained, in writing, from the publisher.

All inquiries should be addressed to ICS Books, Inc., 1370 E. 86th Place, Merrillville, IN 46410

Published by: **Printed in the U.S.A.**
ICS BOOKS, Inc.
1370 E. 86th Place   Cover illustration by
Merrillville, IN 46410   Demetrius Saulsberry
800-541-7323

Co-Published in Canada by:
Vanwell Publishing LTD
1 Northrup Crescent
St. Catharines, Ontario
L2M 6P5
800-661-6136

Library of Congress Cataloging-in-Publication Data
Forgey, William. W, 1942-
Dieter's little book of wisdom / by William Forgey.
p.   cm.
ISBN 1-57034-047-1
1. Weight loss-- Quotations, maxims, etc. I Title.
RM222.2.F675   1996
613.2'5--dc20   96-22509
                                                 CIP

Introduction

During my six years of practice as an emergency room physician and twenty years in family practice, I have routinely had to help people undo the damage done by carelessness, poor habits, and random acts of fate. While we can't help those random acts of fate, we can eliminate a lot of the grief in our lives by some simple preventive measures.

While my book *The Doctor's Little Book of Wisdom* covered all aspects of healthcare and safety issues, amongst the most favorable comments from readers were those relating to hints concerning the problems of weight loss and physical fitness.

For these are the problems that face all of us, all of the time. There is no getting away from it, our constant battle to maintain health is very often related to the food surrounding us—frequently in a negative way.

The menus offered in restaurants and fast-food chains are clogging the arteries of the nation and turning us into a country of behemoths. But there is hope.

National awareness, and an interest in expanding their market share, has caused nearly every fast-food chain to include salad bars and low-fat, low-cholesterol items on their menus. However, you still have to stare at pictures of meat dripping with cheese when you poke your head inside their doors.

The temptations are all around us, but the answers are also there. The answers include realizing the importance of committing yourself to a lifestyle change; knowing that exercise is important, but realizing that you cannot possibly exercise hard enough to make up for high fat diets; and becoming aware of the many delicious healthy snack foods and meals that are possible. The answer also includes knowing you are not alone in this struggle.

There are organizations, both commercial and nonprofit, support groups, and a vast literature of recipes and diet suggestions. This book hopes to be a motivator. Perhaps for yourself or a friend. I hope it helps making a meaningful lifestyle change a little easier. It's never too soon or too late to make this change.

Best wishes for a long and healthy life.
William W. Forgey, M.D.

1. A proper diet works only by developing new habits and tastes.

2. When something is eating you, don't eat to make up for it.

3.   "Low fat" and "low cholesterol"
     do not mean "low calorie."

4.   Exercise both your body and your
      restraint.

5.   Self-restraint when eating is a form of
      self-empowerment.

6. A Kentucky Fried Chicken Rotisserie Gold® white quarter would require one hour of brisk walking to work off. Remove the skin and you could do it in 36 minutes.

7. Driving a motorcycle is almost as strenuous as playing volleyball (204 cal/hour versus 210 cal/hour).

8. You'd have to play volleyball for over 2½ hours to burn off the calories consumed eating two slices of a Dominos® deluxe 12" pizza.

9. Chew slowly and thoroughly—
savor every bite.

10. If you crave cheese, try a light sprinkle
of grated Parmesan cheese for flavor
and the lowest possible additional fat.

11.   All oils are liquid fat.

12.   You can lose weight simply by eliminating any oily or deep-fried food from your diet.

13.   You can lose weight simply by eliminating alcohol from your diet.

14.   Ditto for snacks and non-diet drinks.

15. A Long John Silver's Chicken Planks® dinner would require ten miles to walk off—that's a mighty long plank!

16. All change is stressful at first—
     it disrupts the familiar patterns of life.

17. Disgust motivates change, but fear
     seldom does.

18. If you can't be a vegetarian, then eat a vegetarian.
—Dr. William Castelli, Framingham Heart Study.

19. Like little batteries, calories are stored energy.

20. A calorie is the amount of energy required to raise the temperature of one liter (about one quart) of water one degree Celsius.

21. Sometimes comprehensive diet changes are easier than moderate ones.

22. Don't smoke just to avoid gaining weight.

23.   Over ⅓ of children are overweight.

24.   Adults only 5% overweight are 30% more likely to have heart attacks.

25.   Adults 30% overweight are over 300% more likely to have heart attacks.

26. People are paid an average of $1,000 less per year for each pound they are overweight.

27. If you reduce fat consumption from 40% of calories to 10% of total calories, you can eat ⅓ more food yet take in the same number of calories.

28.   Each time you lose and regain weight, your metabolism slows.

29.   If you reduce food intake by 25%, your metabolism may slow down 20 to 25%.

30.   Reduced metabolism causes a "plateau," weight loss grinds to a halt.

31. The more your weight fluctuates, the higher your risk of heart disease.

32.   Maintain your intake of carbohydrates and reduce fat to maintain your metabolic rate.

33.   One-and-a-half ounces of potato chips have as many calories as one twelve-ounce baked potato.

34.   Eating multiple small meals a day is better than eating fewer large ones.

35. Don't attempt to diet by reducing the amount of food you eat, but by changing the food itself.

36. When dieting, your body first loses fat from areas where you last put it on.

37. In countries where less fat is consumed, there is much less breast cancer.

38. Non-vegetarian women have 50% higher levels of estrogen than vegetarians.

39. High estrogen levels may further the growth of many breast tumors.

40.   Fat is an acquired taste.

41.   Skim milk at first tastes watery; it tastes normal within a few weeks.

42.   Once you are used to skim milk, whole milk tastes too rich.

43. The four basic flavors are salty, sweet, sour, and bitter.

44. Try exploring bitter and sour tastes, along with salty and sweet.

45. Besides flavors, there are also textures to experiment with.

46. The texture to minimize is oily.

47. While possibly stressful at first, comprehensive changes in lifestyle can be easier to maintain as they break you out of your routine which was just making you fat anyway.

48. Pay more attention to what you should be doing than what you shouldn't be doing.

49. Being lonesome is bad for your health.

50. Social bonding is good for health.

51. Teach others that your low fat, low sugar diet can be wonderful.

52. Always eat one meal a day with your family. If this is impossible, do it at least once a week.

53. When eating eggs, avoid the yolk.

54.   Ditto for cooking with eggs.

55.   Use olive oil if you must cook with oil.

56.   Poach fish, rather than frying.

57.   When cooking meats, broil to decrease grease content.

58.   Charred meat causes increased risk of colon cancer.

59.   Drink eight ounces of water daily.

60.   Take an aspirin every day.

61.   Take vitamin E every day.

62.   Never take megadoses of vitamins.

63. Exercise for ½ hour at least three times a week.

64. Encourage a friend to exercise with you.

65. Never salt your food without tasting it first.

66. Never salt your food regardless.

67. Avoid food preserved with nitrites.

68. When eating out, go for the salad bar.

69. At the salad bar, avoid the creamed, cheesy, or greasy items.

70. Avoid constipation by drinking a warm and cold beverage each morning. Answer nature's call when you feel the urge—don't suppress it. And add fruit and bulk to your diet.

71. If you gain ten pounds of weight, this results in forty additional pounds of stress on your knees.

72. Women with tender breasts should avoid caffeine, nicotine, and chocolate—all aggravate fibrocystic breast development.

73. If breasts become tender during or just before your period, avoid salt to help reduce fluid retention.

74. When choosing meat, remember that "select" contains 15 to 20% fat, "choice" has 30 to 40% fat, and "prime" is 40 to 45% fat by weight.

75. Lean pieces can be cut from the fat, unless the portion is marbled.

76. Read labels—take time to compute
     the amounts of fat and cholesterol you
     are eating.

77. Your total fat intake should be less than
     30% of the calories you are eating.

78. Saturated fat should be less than 10% of
     your daily calorie intake.

79.   Cholesterol intake should be less than 300 mg per day.

80.   One 12-oz. can of soft drink has ten teaspoons of sugar.

81.   Alcohol is high in calories and suppresses your body's ability to burn fat.

82. You don't even know what you're missing until you reduce your salt intake. Salt disguises many subtle and wonderful flavors.

83. Eat only in the kitchen or dining room—not wandering around the house or in front of the TV.

84. Don't keep high fat foods around the house.

85. Divide food into smaller portions—eat slices of a pear rather than the whole thing at once.

86. Eat breakfast.

87. Need a snack? One half a banana frozen on a stick makes a perfect Popsickle.

88.   A tablespoon of trimmed chicken fat eliminates 115 calories and 13 grams of fat ($\frac{1}{3}$ of it saturated fat).

89.   Eliminating a tablespoon of half and half from three cups of coffee per day will save you over five pounds of weight gain a year (and possible heart bypass surgery).

90. Commercially ground turkey
     and chicken frequently includes
     fatty skin. Grind it yourself and
     throw away the skin.

91. Longer, slower exercise uses body fat as fuel, while intense exercise uses carbohydrates. It's easier to lose weight with low intensity exercise.

92.   Moderate exercise increases resting metabolism, while intense exercise lowers it.

93.   If you can't talk comfortably while exercising, then you're overdoing it.

94.   Benefit is a more powerful motivation than fear.

95. Make your diet a simple one.

96. Choose a diet that predicts your losses accurately enough that you can follow and confirm your goals week by week.

97. Diet should not be all or nothing.

98. Shish kabob vegetables after marinating them in vegetable broth, lemon juice, and herbs.

99. Make a crust for a vegetable pie by pressing cooked, sticky short grain brown rice into the pie plate.

100. Or try a mashed potato crust.

101. Getting through the day is more important than reaching long-term goals.

102. Water chestnuts are low in calories and make good, crunchy additions to salads.

103. A common reaction to emotional pain is smoking, eating, and drinking.

104. If your best friends are cigarettes, bottles of booze, or piles of food, you will need the support of other friends to control your destiny.

105. Don't think people misunderstand how hard it is to change dietary habits—it's difficult, and they will acknowledge your accomplishment.

106. People commenting on how much weight you've lost is an indication of how much they respect the challenge that you've met.

107. To attempt a diet and to fail is not a disgrace, but rather another battle ribbon in the war of survival.

108. Peanuts are very high in fat and should be avoided as a snack item.

109. Being compulsive is human; controlling it is divine.

110. Just try changing the way you live one day at a time.

111. Giving advice to those not asking for it may only aggravate their feelings about their lifestyle.

112. Lifestyle change frequently requires you look elsewhere.

113.   When your current situation causes
       discomfort, it's time to make a change.

114.   While change is not easy, it's better
       than settling for the discomfort of the
       present situation.

115.   It is natural to desire change and to
       resist change simultaneously.

116. "Homeostasis works to keep things as they are, even if they aren't very good."
—George Leonard

117. Change a vegetable side dish into a main dish by increasing the number of components and adding a flavorful, vegetable-based sauce.

118. You are what you eat.

119. Eat with knowledge.

120. Your mouth can always consume more calories than you can exercise off.

121. Exercise moderation.

122. Japanese noodles are usually fat-free.

123. Avoid non-dairy soy cheese; too much fat and too many calories.

124. Consider flavoring salads with balsamic or herbal vinegars, but avoid adding oil.

125. Top a baked potato with lemon juice and freshly ground black pepper.

126. Bagels with sugar-free jam are a good low-calorie snack.

127. Hungry? Try steamed vegetables with fat-free dressing.

128. Fresh fruits and vegetables are beneficial snack items.

129. For a snack, consider nonfat yogurt.

130. When eating nonfat yogurt, check its total calorie content.

131. Anyone can lose weight; the problem is keeping it off.

132. Being fat is a form of disease, not a human failing.

133. An Egg McMuffin® fuels 1½ hours of vigorous gardening.

134. An Egg McMuffin® three times a week will add eleven pounds to your body in a year.

135. A normal weight person has 25 to 35 billion fat cells, while an obese person has 50 to 150 billion fat cells.

136. When you lose weight, your fat cells shrink but they do not disappear.

137. During periods of weight gain, fat cells can increase their diameters twenty-fold.

138. Even if you have failed many times to lose weight, you can still succeed the next time you try.

139. Rice cakes and sugar-free jelly or jam is a good low-calorie, fat-free fare.

140. Cut down your fat intake. You can eat more food and still lose weight.

141. One pound of pure dietary fat contains 4,082 calories.

142. One pound of sugar contains 1,497 calories.

143. One pound of dietary protein contains 1,814 calories.

144. It's easier to lose weight by counting the grams of fat than counting calories.

145. Light-meat turkey and chicken have much less fat than dark meat.

146. Skinless dark-meat chicken has 8.3 grams of total fat. The same amount of white-meat chicken contains 3.8 grams.

147. To decrease gas problems with bean dishes, soak overnight or parboil and discard the water.

148. Saturated fats cause heart disease, but all fats cause obesity.

149. One hundred percent of margarine calories are fat.

150. The percent of calories from fat in whole milk is 49%, 2% milk still has 37%, but skim milk reduces fat to only 4%.

151. Fiber is present only in plants.

152. High levels of insulin stimulate hunger.

153. Eating sugar increases blood insulin levels.

154. High fiber foods seem to reduce blood levels of insulin.

155. Government guidelines recommend an intake of 20 to 30 grams of fiber per day, but the average American diet includes only 12 grams of fiber per day.

156. If you eat too many calories in a day, you end up storing the excess as fat.

157. When a food package indicates calorie and fat content, watch serving size, not package size.

158. During periods of starvation, your resting metabolic rate can drop.

159. Use fat-free tortilla chips and homemade tomato salsa for a low-calorie snack.

160. Refrigerate soups after cooking so that excess fat can be scraped off the top.

161. Fig bars have less fat than chocolate chip cookies, (but a similar amount of calories).

162. Use mustard, not mayonnaise.

163. A McDonald's Biscuit w/Sausage and Egg® requires five miles of walking to wear off.

164. Two slices of a Pizza Hut Thin 'n' Crispy® medium supreme pizza weekly and you risk adding six pounds per year. Make that a pan pizza and add 7½ pounds.

165. You would have to go 3½ miles to burn off the calories from eating six pieces (one order) of Chicken McNuggets®.

166. Exercise helps give you resolve to skip unnecessary calories.

167. Use stairs rather than take an elevator, or get off three floors away from your destination.

168. Park further from a store or office entrance than necessary.

169. Walk whenever possible.

170. Bring the groceries in from the car one bag at a time to increase your activity level.

171. Increase housework.

172. Dancing burns more calories than chopping firewood.

173. Walking at a rate of three miles per hour burns about 300 calories every hour.

174. You need to walk about 5½ miles to purge the calories of one Wendy's® baked potato with cheese.

175.   A plain baked potato with skin would
       get you two and one-fourth miles.

176.   A boiled potato without skin would
       power you about a mile.

177. Pause for several minutes—count them—before reaching for seconds.

178. Put down your fork between bites.

179. Relax before eating.

180. Leave the table as soon as you are full.

181. Set realistic weight loss goals.

182. Don't leave food items out where they will tempt you.

183. Don't let a setback in your weight-loss program derail your attempts—just start again immediately.

184. By slowing down your rate of
eating, you will enjoy your food
more and eat less of it before
you realize you are no longer
hungry.

185. Do not eat to relieve stress or depression.

186. Develop a plan for losing weight.

187. Eat with your non-dominate hand.

188. Meat and dairy products provide the bulk of dietary saturated fat *and* sodium in the American diet.

189. High-fat diets have been implicated as a causative factor in stroke, high blood pressure, adult-onset diabetes, certain cancers, and gallbladder disorders.

190.   Calories from fat: butter, 100%; avocado, 81%; whole milk, 49%; and 2% milk, 37%.

191.   The body makes all the cholesterol it requires—no additional intake is ever necessary.

192.   Starvation dieting is an unnatural act. Your body will fight every ounce.

193. The most important aspect of losing weight is motivation.

194. Expect to fail and you will.

195. If you fail to lose weight, you are using the wrong plan.

196. A good program results in one
pound of weight loss per week.

197. Consistency in weight loss is more important than the amount per week.

198. Enthusiastically review your weight-loss goals on a daily basis.

199. Constantly conjure up a mental image of how you *wish* to look.

200. Get elated about your new lifestyle. Envision how your new body will appear every day.

201. Consistency is more important than swiftness.

202. Make lifestyle changes that come the easiest for you.

203. Visualize how great you'll look and feel when your goals are met.

204. Look forward to wearing horizontal clothing patterns again.

205. Before you even start your lifestyle change, write down everything you eat during a two-week period.

206. Periodic diaries of all the food you eat will keep you honest.

207. Set intermediate goals with non-caloric rewards as they are achieved.

208. Make your goal more important to you than eating certain foods.

209. Two Arby® potatoes cakes (one serving)
      requires one hour of tennis to neutralize
      the calories you just ate.

210. Would you prefer an order of Arby®
      curly fries? Then spend 1½ hours
      playing tennis.

211. If you plateau your weight loss,
      increase your exercise and replace more
      of your diet with vegetables.

212. If you fail with your lifestyle change, each additional effort will provide you with better habits and help ingrain them.

213. You are better exercising moderately daily than too vigorously less often.

214. Check with your doctor before starting any exercise program.

215. The more weight you have to lose, the more difficult it may seem, but the faster the pounds drop.

216. Ten minutes of walking per day eliminate five pounds of fat in a year.

217. If an increased speed of travel causes loss of efficiency, then more calories are burnt for the same distance.

218. Swimming at 25 yards per minute consumes five calories per minute, while racing at 40 yards per minute consumes an astonishing eleven calories a minute.

219. Decrease your television time to avoid food commercials and increase the opportunity for exercise.

220. Replace one hour of TV with walking and lose 2½ pounds of fat per month.

221. If you're sitting around, it's easy to think about food—Get up, get active.

222. Learn to play—it burns calories.

223. Giving up sugar and fried food
decreases your appetite.

224. Ketogenic diets are: The Atkins Diet
The Drinking Man's Diet (high fat, low
carbohydrate), and The Pennington
Diet (high protein, low carbohydrate),
and starvation.

225. Ketogenic diets should only be undertaken with medical supervision.

226. The Pritikin Diet is a high carbohydrate, low fat diet.

227. If you can stay on them, unbalanced diets work.

228. Nuts and avocados are high in vegetable oils, but are cholesterol-free.

229. Vegetable oils are a source of essential fatty acids and vitamin A.

230. Consume increased amounts of fresh fruits and vegetables.

231. Avoid fried foods.

232. Don't force yourself to eat more when you are full.

233. Don't clean someone else's plate.

234. Don't sample foods while you are cooking.

235. Leave the table as soon as you are finished eating.

236. Have a conversation before taking seconds.

237. If you are a strict vegetarian, include plenty of whole grains (such as brown rice and whole wheat) and legumes (nuts, peas, and beans) to obtain all essential amino acids.

238. Getting slightly drunk adds at least 600 calories to your day—a real drunken blast, several thousand.

239. When boiling vegetables, minimize the boiling time and save the water for soup stock.

240. The more muscle you have, the more fat you can burn.

241. If you wish to increase your exercise, increase the time, not the intensity.

242. Get enough sleep every night.

243. The New Four Foods Group concept diet consists of five or more servings of whole grains, three or more servings of vegetables, two or three servings of legumes or soy products, three or more fruits and other foods if desired as condiments or extras.

244. Use spices as flavor enhancers instead of fats.

245. Use a hot sauce or a curry for a low-fat flavor variation.

246. A tablespoon of oil contains 13.6 grams of fat or 122 calories.

247. Sourdough, French, and pita breads are fat-free (see *Cooking the Sourdough Way* by Scott Power, ICS Books, 1995, for a variety of health recipes).

248. One cup of fresh snow can replace an egg when mixed with batter just prior to baking or grilling (an old Appalachian Mountaineer trick).

249. To avoid butter or margarine, top your pancakes with authentic maple syrup, pure fruit syrup, applesauce or stewed apples.

250. When cooking cereals, add extra water and cook longer—this makes them creamier without adding milk.

251. Each pound of muscle you add to your body uses fifty calories a day just to stay alive.

252. Try salsa as a salad dressing.

253. One beer a day adds one pound of fat in a month.

254. One light beer a day adds ¾ pound, and one nonalcoholic beer, ½ a pound of fat per month.

255. Eight ounces of Tang® a day could result in ten pounds of fat in a year.

256. A Mars® bar a day adds 1½ pounds of fat in a month.

257. One cup of All Bran® has slightly less fat and 12 times the fiber of a cup of Cheerios®, but over twice the calories. The secret ingredient in Cheerios® is lots of low-calorie air.

258. Canned beans and franks have twice the calories and fat of canned beef stew.

259. Canned beef stew has three times the saturated and total fat as canned refried beans.

260. One cup of fish Creole has ⅕ th the fat and ½ the calories of corned beef hash.

261. Frying fish rather than broiling yields ten times the fat and twice the calories.

262. You'd have to chop firewood for one hour and 18 minutes to burn off one regular Arby® Roast Beef sandwich.

263. Or briskly walk one hour and 25 minutes to consume the calories in one Whopper®.

264. Eating one Mars® bar would require over one hour of volleyball playing to avoid weight gain.

265. Three ounces of Shoney's® french fries a week would add 2½ lbs of fat to your body per year.

266. One Sausage McMuffin w/Egg® per week would add 5½ lbs to your weight in a year—one a day, 38 pounds!

267. Dip your bread into soup, not butter.

268. Use a barbecue sauce in place of butter for corn on the cob.

269. Substitute cocktail sauce for tartar sauce.

270. Briefly refrigerate gravy to scrape off the solid fat before reheating and serving.

271. Instead of thickening gravy with flour and fat, use cornstarch.

272. The very leanest cuts of beef with all fat removed still have a *minimum* of 29% of their calories from fat.

273. White chicken meat with the skin removed still gets 19% of its calories from fat.

274. Once less chocolate shake per week is four less pounds per year.

275. One small three-ring pretzel per day adds a pound a year.

276. For each small pretzel that you eat, walk three minutes.

277. Nothing will ever taste as good as thin looks.

278. The best tasting soups are a combination of vegetables and a starch or protein—and low-fat, low-calorie choices are abundant.

279. Use nonfat buttermilk as the base for any creamy dressing.

280. Ground nuts can provide less oil than an oil-based dressing for salads..

281. Use leftover pasta as part of a stir-fry.

282. If you insist on oil for a salad dressing, simply spritz a little from a spray bottle.

283. Try seasoned rice vinegar from an Oriental market for a low-calorie, yet tasty, salad dressing.

284. For a bread topping, use small amounts of nonfat yogurt.

285. Enhance interest in vegetable dishes by choosing an exotic or less well-known variety.

286. Try cooking grains (such as barley, rice, buckwheat) in a vegetable broth.

287. Use crushed corn flakes on top of a casserole instead of grated cheese or nuts.

288. Celebrating with an extra serving or with forbidden food doesn't mean you have failed your diet.

289. Dilute the fat content of a meat loaf or hamburger with cooked rice, other vegetables, or mixing in mashed potatoes.

290. Buy tortillas made without shortening.

291. Use meat only as a flavoring and not as the main ingredient of a dish.

292. Use a flour tortilla instead of pie crust for baking pot pies.

293. Be careful with those turkey tubes—some chicken and turkey hot dogs have as much fat as the beef and pork types.

294.   Skinless turkey has ⅓ less fat than
        skinless chicken.

295.   Try cooking vegetables in a fruit juice.

296.   Use garlic powder as a sprinkle on leafy
        vegetables in place of dressing.

297.   Improve any bland, nonfat food with a
        dash of pepper sauce.

298. Try various pepper sauces in small amounts to enhance stews and soups.

299. For a change, replace lettuce with Vidalia onion slices in any dish.

300. Replace candy with dried fruits.

301. Snack on fruit and raw vegetables, not starch or sugar.

302. Top a baked potato with a dab of cold, mashed sweet potato.

303. Make a salad sandwich.

304. Buy Scandinavian-style crackers (such as Wasabrod)—very low in fat.

305. Make popcorn with an air-popper.

306. Try toasting oats or chickpeas on a cookie sheet for crunchy snacks.

307. Try slicing fresh mushrooms and serving with balsamic vinaigrette.

308. Cookies are a more common binge food than hard candies.

309. Chocolates are a more disastrous binge food than cookies.

310. A friend who brings binge food as a present is a Unabomber in disguise.

311. A tablespoon of butter contains 108 calories.

312. Each ounce of beef fat removed from your diet saves your consuming 216 calories and six grams of saturated fat.

313. California avocados have 51 calories per ounce, while Florida avocados only have 31 calories per ounce. The Florida variety also has much less sodium.

314. A canned fig has fewer calories than a fresh fig (25 vs 37) or a dried fig (at 48 calories each).

315. The amount of calories burned by various activities frequently depend upon your weight and the intensity of the exercise.

316. A 140-pound person would burn 87 calories in 30 minutes walking at a leisurely two miles per hour, while a 180 pound individual would burn 105 calories.

317. When walking for exercise, the surface greatly influences the amount of energy consumed.

318. When walking on markedly rough surfaces, slower speeds will compensate for the surface difference.

319. A 140-pound individual walking on a hard surface at 3½ mph burns 276 calories per hour, while the same pace on grass consumes 336 calories.

320. A 180-pound individual walking on a hard surface at 3½ mph burns 325 calories per hour on asphalt or 714 calories/hour on hard snow.

321. If you ate one regular Dairy Queen® vanilla ice cream cone, swim 1100 yards to lose the fat; if dipped in chocolate, 1600 yards.

322. You need to swim for two hours to eliminate the calories from a Burger King Whopper®; Whopper double beef with cheese®, make that three hours six minutes—and you had better wait an hour before entering the water.

323. A Burger King Ocean Catch® fish fillet will cost you 1¾ hours of continuous work on the stationary bike to burn up the 479 calories you just ate. The same serving size poached would only be 22 minutes.

324. A Big Mac® would take 2⅓ hours of continuous volleyball to nullify.

325. A McDonald's® breakfast burrito provides the calories for 50 minutes of brisk walking.

326. Feel like a long walk? You could go over five miles on the calories in two slices of a Pizza Hut® medium cheese hand-tossed pizza.

327. A Taco Bell® Mexican pizza requires 5½ miles of walking to erase.

328. A small Wendy's® chocolate frosty will fuel 47 minutes of vigorous tennis.

329. A Wendy's® junior cheeseburger is equal to one hour on a treadmill at a vigorous clip.

330. One Wendy's® baked potato with cheese requires 2½ hours of driving a motorcycle to prevent adding additional weight.

331. The difference between a side salad with diet dressing vs. regular dressing is about 52 additional minutes of vigorous workout on a treadmill.

332. Eating is frequently ritualistic.
Change your patterns.

333. Believe in it before you try it.

334. Avoid guilt trips.

335. Suffering motivates change.

336. Fear does not motivate change.

337. A teaspoon of any cooking oil has 45 calories and five grams of fat.

338. Use cooking oil sprays rather than oil.

339. In place of ice cream, use frozen nonfat yogurt.

340. Rather than sour cream, try plain nonfat yogurt.

341. Take a hint from Weight Watchers®: lose weight with a friend.

342. Take a hint: also exercise with a friend.

343. "Some habits must be eased downstairs
a step at a time"
—Mark Twain

344. The normal cake with the lowest fat is
angel food.

345. Use a mixture of vegetable broth and a little cornstarch in place of oil for a salad dressing.

346. Use dried soup mix as a topping for a baked potato instead of sour cream or butter.

347. You must rely on the support of friends to help you get through life—not a dependency on alcohol, drugs, TV, or food.

348. You would have to canoe aggressively for over an hour to burn the calories of one Shoney's® All American Burger.

349. Or walk 5½ miles.

350. Because meals are important social
      forms of interacting with others,
      structure them to aid your dietary goals.

351. Bass and sardines are high in fat, while the lowest fat levels in fish are found in cod, haddock, and yellowfin tuna.

352. Three ounces of cooked herring has less than one gram of fat and only eight percent of its calories from fat.

353. Cooked freshwater bass has four grams of fat per three ounce serving and 29 percent of its calories from fat.

354. Never eat while standing.

355. Never eat anything larger than your head.

356. Use nonfat monterey jack, cheddar, Swiss, or American cheeses for fewer calories and lower fat content.

357. Legumes are high in fiber, protein and many other nutrients—and low in fat.

358. Eat one part legumes to three parts grains to provide the proper mix of protein.

359. Typical legumes are beans, peas, soybeans and lentils.

360. To speed up cooking beans, use a pressure cooker.

361. Hunger can lead to rebound eating. This adds more calories than were lost during the entire starvation period.

362. Slipping from a diet is not failure; it's a part of normal life. Don't use slippage as an excuse to abandon your lifestyle changes.

363. Eat whole grain rather than refined white flour to increase B and E vitamins and add fiber to your diet.

364. No one wants to hire you when you are fat—and wages prove it.

365. First help yourself, then help others.

366. Place your snack money in a new clothes fund.

367. If you are overweight, there is a reason for it—and most of the reason is mental, not metabolic.

368. Depending upon your weight, you would have to walk at least 35 miles to lose one pound.

The Little Books of Wisdom Series

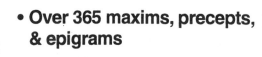

- **Over 365 maxims, precepts, & epigrams**

- **160 pages** • **6 x 4 1/2**

- **Each Only $5.95** ($7.95 Canada)

Parent's Little Book of Wisdom by Tilton / Gray ISBN 1-57034-039-0
Writer's Little Book of Wisdom by John Long ISBN 1-57034-037-4
Bachelor's Little Book of Wisdom by David Scott ISBN 1-57034-038-2
Traveler's Little Book of Wisdom by Forgey, M.D. / Scott ISBN 1-57034-036-6
Canoeist's Little Book of Wisdom by Cliff Jacobson ISBN 1-57034-040-4
Teacher's Little Book of Wisdom by Bob Algozzine ISBN 1-57034-017-X
Doctor's Little Book of Wisdom by William W. Forgey M.D. ISBN 1-57034-016-1
Camping's Little Book of Wisdom by David Scott ISBN 0-934802-96-3
Handyman's Little Book of Wisdom by Bob Algozzine ISBN 1-57034-046-3
Dieter's Little Book of Wisdom by William W. Forgey M.D. ISBN 1-57034-047-1
Musician's Little Book of Wisdom by Scott Power ISBN 1-57034-048-X

For a FREE catalog of all ICS BOOKS titles Call 1-800-541-7323
e-Mail us at **booksics@aol.com** or look for us at **http://www.onlinesports.com/ics**